Better Health with Dr Das

A Doctor's Easy Guide to Understanding & Managing HIGH BLOOD PRESSURE

Dr Prabhat Das

MD, PhD, FACP

Disclaimer

This book is intended solely for educational and informational purposes. It is not meant to replace personal medical advice, diagnosis, or treatment. Although I am a licensed physician, reading this book does not establish a doctor–patient relationship. Each individual's health condition, medical history, and risk factors are unique. Any medical decision should be made in partnership with your own healthcare professional who understands your specific situation. Medical science is continually advancing. New research and updated guidelines may lead to changes in recommendations over time.

Paperback ISBN: 978-1-971672-02-1
eBook ISBN: 978-1-971672-03-8

Printed in the United States of America

Why I Wrote This BOOK

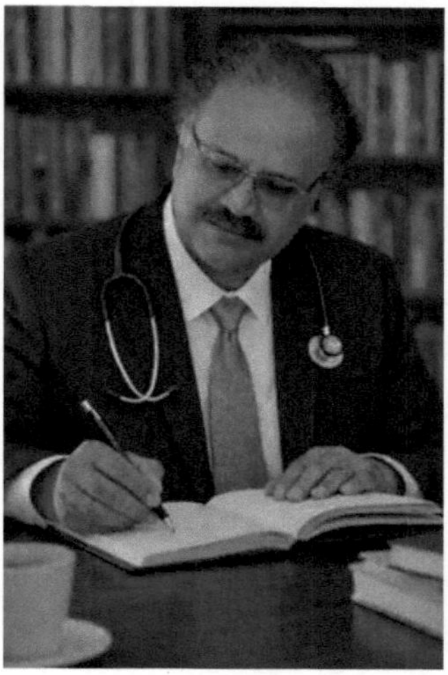

I am Dr Prabhat Das, MD, PhD, and a Fellow of the American College of Physicians. I am trained in Internal Medicine, Pulmonary Diseases, and Critical Care. My medical journey began in India and has continued in the United States for more than thirty-five years. During these decades, my work has taken me from quiet clinic visits to busy hospital wards, from routine checkups to moments when quick, careful decisions truly mattered. Through it all, medicine has never felt like just a profession to me. It has been a lifelong commitment to learning, caring, and standing beside people during some of the most vulnerable moments of their lives.

Among all the conditions I have seen over the years, high blood pressure stands out in a troubling way. Not because it is rare, but because it is common, silent, and often ignored. Many patients sit across from me and say, "Doctor, I feel fine." Most of the time, they truly do. That is exactly why high blood pressure is so dangerous. It quietly causes damage while daily life goes on uninterrupted. People remain busy with work, family, responsibilities, and stress. When nothing hurts, health is easy to postpone.

This book was written to change that pattern. My goal is to make high blood pressure understandable, less frightening, and truly manageable. When people understand what their blood pressure numbers mean, fear decreases and confidence grows. And when confidence grows, good habits are far more likely to last.

This book is not meant to replace your doctor. It is meant to help you become an informed and confident partner in your own care. Knowledge allows better conversations, better questions, and better decisions. Whether you are newly diagnosed, have lived with high blood pressure for years, or are simply trying to prevent problems in the future, this book is designed to meet you where you are.

Through the *Better Health with Dr Das* series, I hope to reach people I may never meet in my office. Many individuals live with health concerns, confusion, and quiet anxiety, often without clear and trustworthy guidance. My aim is to explain medical problems in a simple, practical, and honest way, so readers feel informed rather than frightened, and supported rather than overwhelmed.

High blood pressure does not require panic or extreme measures. It requires understanding, patience, and steady care. This book will walk with you, step by step, toward better control and better long-term health.

Table of Contents

Why I Wrote This BOOK v

Chapter 1: Blood Pressure Made Simple 1

Chapter 2: Why Blood Pressure Rises 9

Chapter 3: Essential and Secondary Hypertension 17

Chapter 4: How High Blood Pressure Is Diagnosed 25

Chapter 5: The Damage High Blood Pressure Can Cause 33

Chapter 6: Food, Salt, and Blood Pressure 41

Chapter 7: Lifestyle Habits That Shape Blood Pressure 47

Chapter 8: Medicines Are Needed, When Lifestyle Changes Are Not Enough 53

Chapter 9: Blood Pressure Medications Explained Clearly 59

Chapter 10: Special Situations and Difficult-to-Control Blood Pressure 67

Chapter 11: Your Practical Plan to Control Blood Pressure for Life 73

Chapter 12: Common Myths and Misconceptions About High Blood Pressure 79

Chapter 13: Blood Pressure Across Different Stages of Life 87

Chapter 14: Frequently Asked Questions Patients Ask Their Doctor 93

Chapter 15: Why Many People Hesitate to Start Blood Pressure Medication 99

Chapter 16: Taking Your Blood Pressure Correctly 105

Chapter 17: Conclusion: Final Message to the Reader 113

Thank You and Please Review the Book. 117

Continue your Healthcare Journey 118

Chapter 1
Blood Pressure Made Simple

Blood pressure is often reduced to a routine number. A cuff tightens around the arm, two numbers appear, and the moment passes. For many people, those numbers feel abstract and easy to forget. Yet they quietly reflect how the heart, blood vessels, and vital organs are functioning every day.

Blood pressure is not just a measurement. It is a window into the health of your circulation. It tells us how hard the heart must work, how flexible or stiff the arteries have become, and how much ongoing strain the organs are experiencing. Long before symptoms appear, blood pressure begins to reveal important changes inside the body.

This chapter lays the foundation for everything that follows. Before discussing causes, complications, or treatment, blood pressure itself must feel clear and familiar. When people understand what blood pressure means and why it matters, fear decreases. In its place comes confidence, and confidence leads to better long-term decisions.

One of the most dangerous features of high blood pressure is its silence. Most people feel completely normal, sometimes for many years. Many say, "I feel fine," or "I would know if something was wrong." Unfortunately, blood pressure does not behave that way. The body adapts quietly to higher pressure, even as damage slowly develops in the background.

Understanding blood pressure is the first and most important step toward protecting your health.

What Blood Pressure Really Means

Blood pressure is the force of blood pushing against the walls of the arteries as the heart pumps. The heart acts as a steady pump. The arteries act as flexible tubes that carry blood to every part of the body.

Each heartbeat pushes blood forward under pressure. That pressure is essential for life. Without it, oxygen and nutrients would not reach the brain, kidneys, muscles, and other organs. A temporary rise in blood pressure is normal and healthy. It happens during physical activity, emotional stress, excitement, or pain.

Problems arise when blood pressure stays high most of the time, even when the body is at rest. Instead of rising and falling naturally, pressure remains elevated day after day. This creates constant strain on the heart and blood vessels.

Over time, this strain leads to physical changes. The heart must work harder with every beat. Arteries become thicker and less flexible. These changes develop slowly and often without warning signs. High blood pressure is therefore not a sudden event, but a long-term process.

Blood pressure is not just a number. It represents ongoing stress inside the body.

Understanding the Two Blood Pressure Numbers

Blood pressure is written as two numbers, such as 120 over 80. Each number reflects a different phase of the heartbeat.

The top number, called systolic pressure, measures the force in the arteries when the heart contracts and pushes blood forward.

The bottom number, called diastolic pressure, measures the force in the arteries when the heart relaxes between beats and fills with blood.

A simple way to remember this is:

Systolic pressure reflects the push.

Diastolic pressure reflects the rest.

Both numbers matter. In younger adults, elevations in either number increases long-term risk. With aging, arteries gradually lose flexibility. As a result, systolic pressure often rises, even if the diastolic number stays normal.

This is why doctors focus on trends over time rather than single reading. One isolated number rarely tells the full story.

How Blood Pressure Is Measured

Blood pressure is measured in millimeters of mercury, written as mm Hg. Although this unit comes from older measuring techniques, it remains the standard used worldwide.

Blood pressure can be measured in several settings:

- In a doctor's office
- At home using a validated monitor
- With ambulatory monitoring over twenty-four hours

Blood pressure naturally changes throughout the day. Activity, stress, pain, caffeine, and even conversation can temporarily raise readings.

Many people experience higher readings in medical settings because of anxiety. This is known as the white coat effect. For this reason, diagnosis is based on repeated measurements taken over time, often including readings taken at home.

Accuracy matters more than speed. Careful measurement prevents both unnecessary treatment and missed diagnosis.

What Is Considered Normal Blood Pressure

In adults, commonly used categories include:

- Normal: systolic below 120 and diastolic below 80
- Elevated: systolic 120 to 129 with diastolic below 80
- High blood pressure stage 1: systolic 130 to 139 or diastolic 80 to 89
- High blood pressure stage 2: systolic 140 or higher or diastolic 90 or higher

These ranges are guides, not rigid labels. Individual goals may vary depending on age, overall health, and associated conditions.

What matters most is the long-term pattern, not a single reading.

Why Blood Pressure Matters

High blood pressure usually causes no symptoms for many years. During this time, strain on the heart and blood vessels continues quietly.

Persistently high pressure can:

- Thicken and stiffen the heart muscle
- Damage artery walls
- Reduce healthy blood flow to vital organs

Because blood pressure fluctuates naturally, correct measurement technique is essential. Sitting calmly, using the proper cuff size, and repeating measurements improve reliability.

Visualizing the heart as a pump and the arteries as flexible tubes helps make sense of everything that follows in this book.

Two Everyday Examples

Example one:

A man measures his blood pressure immediately after climbing stairs. The reading is high and causes concern. Later, after resting and measuring correctly, his readings are lower. The lesson is to focus on proper technique and patterns, not single readings.

Example two:

A woman has high readings in the doctor's office but normal readings at home. Home monitoring confirms her usual blood pressure and prevents unnecessary treatment. The lesson is that setting matters.

Summary

- Blood pressure reflects the force of blood against artery walls
- High blood pressure usually develops slowly and silently
- Systolic and diastolic numbers describe different phases of the heartbeat
- Accurate measurement over time is essential
- Categories guide risk but do not replace individual judgment
- Understanding blood pressure is the foundation of control

Your Practical Action Plan

1. Learn proper blood pressure measurement technique.
2. Measure blood pressure on multiple days, not just once.
3. Record all readings honestly and consistently.
4. Focus on trends rather than individual numbers.
5. Share your readings with your clinician before drawing conclusions.

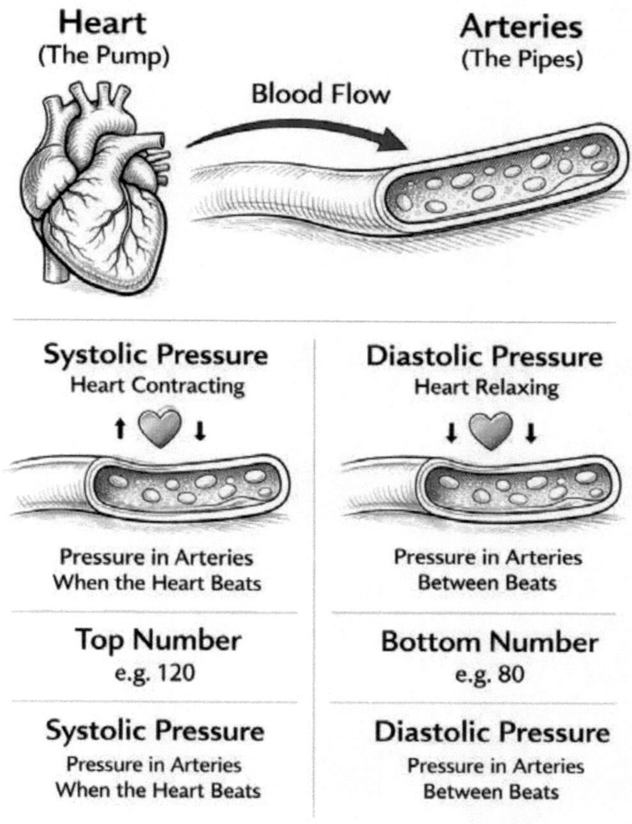

Figure 1.1 Understanding Blood Pressure: Systolic (Bottom)

Transition to Chapter 2

In the next chapter, we will explore why blood pressure rises in the first place and how everyday factors slowly shape those numbers over time.

Chapter 2
Why Blood Pressure Rises

For most people, high blood pressure does not appear suddenly. It develops slowly, often over many years, shaped by age, habits, environment, and internal body changes. Because this rise is gradual, it often goes unnoticed. People feel well, continue their daily routines, and the numbers quietly drift upward in the background.

Understanding why blood pressure rises is essential. Causes point toward solutions. When people understand what is pushing their blood pressure higher, they feel less anxious and more in control. This chapter explains the common forces that raise blood pressure and how they work together over time.

High blood pressure is rarely caused by a single factor. In most cases, several small influences add up gradually. Recognizing these influences early allows timely action and long-term protection.

How Blood Pressure Is Influenced Inside the Body

Blood pressure is mainly determined by two factors. The first is how much blood is flowing through the arteries. The second is how tight or relaxed those arteries are.

If the body holds extra salt and water, blood volume increases. More volume inside the blood vessels leads to higher pressure. If blood vessels remain slightly tightened rather than relaxed, resistance increases. Either change can raise blood pressure. When both occur together over time, blood pressure rises steadily.

These changes usually develop slowly. The body adapts to them and begins to treat higher pressure as normal unless something interrupts the process.

Common Factors That Raise Blood Pressure

In daily life, several factors commonly contribute to rising blood pressure:

- Increasing age
- Family history of high blood pressure
- Excess body weight, especially around the abdomen
- High intake of salt and processed foods
- Low physical activity
- Chronic emotional or work-related stress
- Poor or inconsistent sleep

- Excess alcohol intake

Each of these factors may appear modest on its own. Together, they create a steady workload on the heart and blood vessels. Over time, this workload raises blood pressure.

Many of these factors reinforce each other. Stress can disrupt sleep. Poor sleep can promote weight gain. Weight gain increases blood pressure. Once this cycle begins, it tends to continue unless deliberate changes are made.

Role of Age and Family History

Age plays an important role in blood pressure. As people grow older, arteries gradually lose elasticity. Healthy arteries expand with each heartbeat, absorbing pressure. Stiffer arteries do not expand as easily. The heart must then pump against greater resistance, which raises blood pressure, especially the systolic number.

Family history also matters. If close relatives have high blood pressure, the risk is higher. This does not mean hypertension is unavoidable. It means the body may be more sensitive to salt, weight changes, and stress.

Genetics set the background. Lifestyle determines how strongly that background influences blood pressure. Early awareness allows earlier and more effective prevention.

Salt, Weight, and Modern Lifestyle

Salt has a direct effect on blood pressure. Sodium causes the body to retain water. When extra fluid stays in the bloodstream, pressure inside the arteries rises.

Most people consume more sodium than they realize. Most of the salt comes from packaged foods, restaurant meals, sauces, breads, and processed items rather than from salt added at the table.

Some individuals are salt sensitive. Their kidneys do not remove sodium efficiently, causing fluid retention and higher blood pressure. Salt sensitivity becomes more common with age, kidney disease, diabetes, and strong family history.

Excess body weight raises blood pressure through multiple pathways. A larger body requires more blood flow, increasing heart workload. Fat tissue also alters hormone signals, keeping blood vessels slightly tightened and promoting sodium retention.

Modern life often combines high sodium intake, long sitting hours, reduced movement, shorter sleep, and ongoing stress. Blood pressure gradually reflects this environment, even when no single factor seems extreme.

Stress, Sleep, and Hormonal Effects

Short-term stress causes temporary increases in blood pressure. This is normal and expected. Problems arise when stress becomes chronic.

Chronic stress keeps stress hormones elevated. These hormones tighten blood vessels, increase heart rate, and encourage the body to retain sodium. Blood pressure begins to run higher even at rest.

Sleep plays a critical role. During healthy sleep, blood pressure normally falls. Poor or insufficient sleep disrupts this nightly recovery. Over time, lack of restorative sleep contributes to sustained hypertension.

Understanding these effects helps explain why improving sleep and managing stress are essential parts of blood pressure control.

Two Everyday Examples

Example one:

A man gradually gains weight, eats more packaged foods, and becomes less active over several years. He feels well, but his blood pressure rises slowly into the high range. The lesson is that gradual changes add up.

Example two:

A woman notices mildly elevated readings in her late forties. She reduces sodium intake, walks regularly, improves sleep, and manages stress more intentionally. Her readings stabilize. The lesson is that early correction works.

Summary

- Blood pressure is influenced by blood volume and vessel resistance
- High blood pressure usually develops gradually
- Age and family history increase risk
- Excess salt and weight raise pressure through fluid and hormone effects
- Stress and poor sleep keep blood pressure elevated
- Understanding causes guides effective prevention

WHY BLOOD PRESSURE RISES

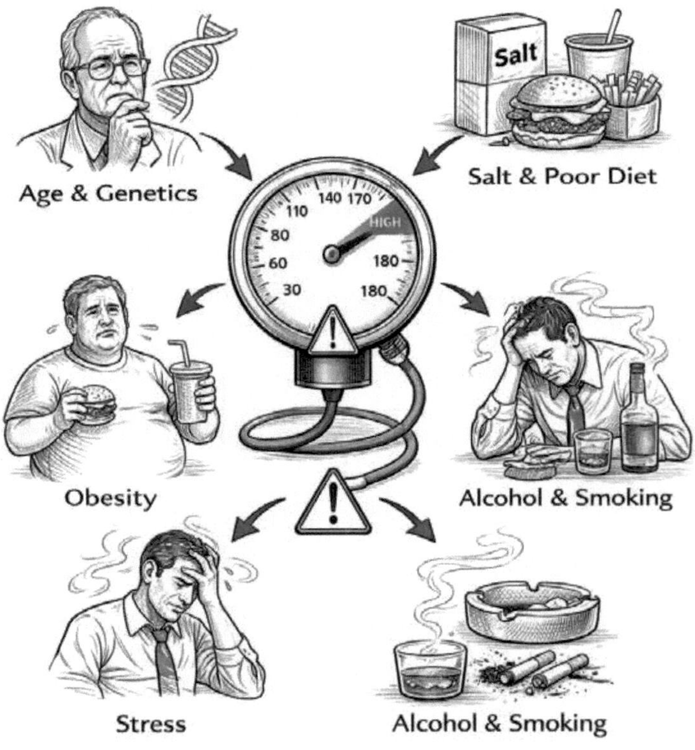
Salt
Age & Genetics
Salt & Poor Diet
110
140 170
HIGH
80
60
180
30
180
Obesity
Alcohol & Smoking
Stress
Alcohol & Smoking

Your Practical Action Plan

1. Identify the two strongest factors influencing your blood pressure.
2. Reduce one major source of excess sodium in your routine.
3. Add regular physical movement that fits your daily life.
4. Protect sleep consistency and quality.
5. Remember that gradual changes produce lasting results.

Transition to Chapter 3

In the next chapter, we will distinguish between essential and secondary hypertension and explain why identifying the type of high blood pressure matters for treatment decisions.

Chapter 3
Essential and Secondary Hypertension

Once high blood pressure is identified, the next important step is understanding what type it is. This distinction shapes everything that follows, from how much testing is needed to how treatment is planned. Not all high blood pressure behaves the same way, and not all of it is managed in the same manner.

Doctors broadly classify high blood pressure into two categories: essential hypertension and secondary hypertension. Most people fall into the first group. A smaller but important number of people fall into the second. Knowing the difference helps avoid unnecessary worry while ensuring that important causes are not missed.

This chapter explains these two types in clear, practical terms and shows why this distinction matters for long-term care.

What Is Essential Hypertension

Essential hypertension, also called primary hypertension, is the most common form of high blood pressure. The vast majority of adults with hypertension have this type.

In essential hypertension, there is no single identifiable cause. Instead, blood pressure rises gradually due to a combination of aging, inherited tendencies, and long-term lifestyle factors. Over time, small influences add up and become significant.

Several processes often occur together:

- Gradual stiffening of arteries with age
- Increased sensitivity to salt
- Slow weight gain
- Reduced physical activity
- Ongoing emotional or mental stress

The body adapts to these changes and begins to accept higher pressure as normal. Unless something interrupts this pattern, elevated blood pressure becomes the new baseline.

Essential hypertension is not mysterious or untreatable. It simply means there is no single switch to turn off. Management focuses on steady control rather than eliminating one cause.

What Is Secondary Hypertension

Secondary hypertension differs in one important way. It is driven by a specific underlying condition or substance. When that cause is identified and addressed, blood pressure often improves significantly and may return to normal.

Secondary hypertension is less common, but it carries special importance because treatment can be targeted. Instead of managing blood pressure indefinitely, doctors may be able to correct or reduce the underlying driver.

This form of hypertension often behaves differently. Blood pressure may rise more suddenly, reach higher levels, or respond poorly to standard treatment. These patterns prompt doctors to look more closely for an underlying cause.

Conditions That Can Raise Blood Pressure

Several medical conditions can directly raise blood pressure by affecting salt balance, hormone levels, or blood vessel tone.

Common examples include:

- Chronic kidney disease
- Narrowing of the arteries supplying the kidneys
- Hormonal disorders that increase fluid retention or vessel tightening
- Sleep apnea, which activates stress responses during sleep
- Thyroid disorders that alter circulation and metabolism

These conditions do not cause high blood pressure quietly over decades. They usually produce patterns that stand out, either by severity, timing, or resistance to treatment.

Recognizing these patterns allows timely evaluation and appropriate care.

Medications and Substances That Increase Blood Pressure

Sometimes high blood pressure is driven not by disease, but by medications or substances that raise pressure as a side effect.

Common contributors include:

- Certain pain relievers when used frequently
- Some cold and allergy medications
- Hormonal treatments
- Excess alcohol intake
- Stimulants and some supplements

This is why a complete medication review is an essential part of blood pressure evaluation. Over-the-counter products and supplements matter just as much as prescription medications.

Changes should never be made abruptly or without guidance. Often, simple adjustments are enough to improve control.

When Doctors Suspect a Secondary Cause

Most people with high blood pressure do not need extensive testing. However, certain patterns suggest that secondary hypertension may be present.

Doctors become more alert when blood pressure:

- Appears suddenly rather than gradually
- Is very high at diagnosis
- Remains uncontrolled despite appropriate treatment
- Occurs at a younger age
- Is associated with abnormal test results

In these situations, targeted evaluation helps identify causes that may be corrected or better managed.

Understanding this process reassures patients that testing is purposeful, not excessive.

Two Everyday Examples

Example one:

A retired teacher develops gradually rising blood pressure over many years. Lifestyle changes help, but medication is eventually needed. No single cause is found. The lesson is that essential hypertension requires steady long-term control.

Example two:

A middle-aged man develops sudden and severe elevation of blood pressure. Further evaluation reveals a kidney-related problem. Treating the underlying condition improves his readings. The lesson is that identifying a cause can change the treatment path.

ESSENTIAL AND SECONDARY HYPERTENSION

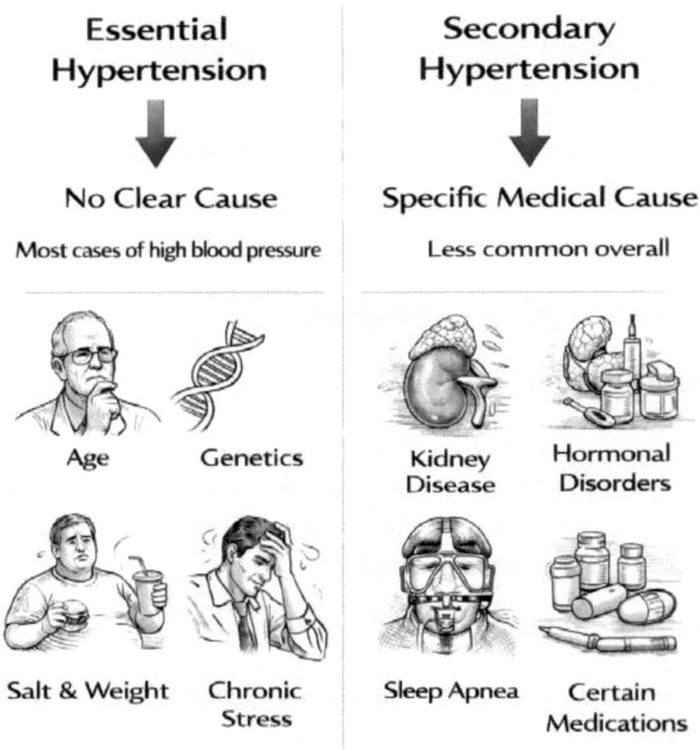

Summary

- High blood pressure is classified as essential or secondary
- Essential hypertension develops gradually from multiple influences
- Secondary hypertension is driven by a specific cause
- Certain medical conditions and substances raise blood pressure
- Unusual patterns prompt further evaluation
- Identifying the type guides effective treatment

Your Practical Action Plan

1. Ask whether your blood pressure rise was gradual or sudden.
2. Review all medications and supplements honestly.
3. Do not fear evaluation when patterns seem unusual.
4. Focus on steady control if hypertension is essential.
5. Support targeted treatment if a secondary cause is identified.

Transition to Chapter 4

In the next chapter, we will focus on how high blood pressure is diagnosed correctly and why careful measurement over time is just as important as the numbers themselves.

Chapter 4
How High Blood Pressure Is Diagnosed

The word diagnosis can sound serious and final. For many people, it brings anxiety even before any discussion begins. When it comes to high blood pressure, however, diagnosis is far less dramatic than it sounds. It simply means answering two essential questions. Are the blood pressure readings truly high, and are they high often enough to matter?

Getting this right is critically important. A rushed diagnosis can lead to unnecessary worry and treatment. A missed diagnosis can allow silent damage to continue unchecked. High blood pressure is not diagnosed in a single visit or from a single reading. It is diagnosed thoughtfully, over time, with care and context.

This chapter explains how blood pressure is diagnosed correctly and why patience and proper technique matter far more than speed.

What Diagnosis Really Means in Hypertension

Unlike many conditions, high blood pressure does not declare itself with symptoms or sudden changes. Diagnosis depends entirely on accurate measurement and interpretation.

Blood pressure naturally fluctuates throughout the day. It rises with activity, stress, pain, and anxiety. It falls with rest and sleep. Because of this normal variability, diagnosis is based on patterns, not isolated numbers.

A good diagnosis answers three questions:

- What are the usual blood pressure levels?
- How consistent are those readings?
- Do they place the person at long-term risk?

Only when these questions are answered clearly does diagnosis become meaningful.

Office Blood Pressure Readings Explained

For most people, blood pressure measurement begins in the doctor's office. These readings are important, but they are rarely the full story.

Many individuals feel anxious in medical settings. Even mild nervousness can activate stress responses that temporarily raise blood pressure. This effect is known as the white coat effect.

Because of this, a single high office reading does not automatically mean hypertension. Doctors look for repeated readings taken properly, often across multiple visits.

Context also matters. Was the patient rushed? In pain? Recently active? Talking during the measurement? All of these factors can influence readings.

Office measurements are best viewed as an initial signal, not a final verdict.

Home Blood Pressure Monitoring

Home blood pressure monitoring has become one of the most valuable tools in modern hypertension care. Measuring blood pressure in a familiar, relaxed environment often provides a more accurate picture of usual levels.

Home monitoring is useful because it:

- Reduces anxiety-related spikes
- Provides multiple readings over several days
- Reveals day-to-day patterns
- Encourages patient understanding and involvement

A common approach is to measure blood pressure in the morning and evening, take two readings each time, and record results for several days.

What matters most is the trend, not the highest or lowest number. A week of home readings often tells a clearer story than a single office visit.

Ambulatory Blood Pressure Monitoring

Ambulatory blood pressure monitoring involves wearing a small device for twenty four hours. The device measures blood pressure periodically during normal daily activities and during sleep.

This method provides information that cannot be obtained otherwise. It is especially helpful when:

- Office and home readings disagree
- Blood pressure varies widely
- White coat or masked hypertension is suspected
- Nighttime blood pressure patterns need evaluation

Blood pressure normally drops during sleep. If it does not, long-term cardiovascular risk may be higher. Ambulatory monitoring helps detect this pattern early and guide treatment more precisely.

Common Errors That Lead to Wrong Diagnosis

Many diagnostic errors occur not because of disease complexity, but because of simple measurement mistakes.

Common errors include:

- Measuring too soon after physical activity
- Using an incorrect cuff size
- Talking during the reading
- Sitting without back or arm support
- Relying on a single measurement

Even small mistakes can raise readings significantly. Correct technique does not need to be perfect. It needs to be consistent.

Learning proper measurement technique protects patients from both overdiagnosis and missed diagnosis.

Excluding Secondary Causes

Once high blood pressure is confirmed, doctors consider whether secondary hypertension may be present, especially when blood pressure behaves unusually.

Further evaluation is more likely when blood pressure:

- Appears at a young age
- Is very high at diagnosis
- Develops suddenly rather than gradually
- Remains uncontrolled despite treatment

Initial evaluation often includes basic blood tests, urine testing, and sometimes an electrocardiogram. Additional tests are guided by findings rather than performed routinely.

The goal is not excessive testing. It is to rule out important and treatable causes when the pattern suggests they may be present.

Two Everyday Examples

Example one: the single reading trap

A man is told his blood pressure is high after one rushed office reading. No repeat measurements are taken. Later, careful home monitoring shows normal readings. A premature diagnosis could have been avoided.

Example two: the hidden risk

A woman's office readings appear normal, but home monitoring reveals consistently elevated blood pressure. Early diagnosis allows timely lifestyle changes before silent damage occurs.

Summary

- High blood pressure is diagnosed over time, not in a single visit
- Office readings are important but often incomplete
- Home monitoring provides real-world patterns
- Ambulatory monitoring reveals daily and nighttime behavior
- Measurement errors can lead to misdiagnosis
- Secondary causes are considered when patterns are unusual

Your Practical Action Plan

1. Learn correct blood pressure measurement technique and use it consistently.
2. Do not rely on a single reading to draw conclusions.
3. Use home monitoring when recommended.
4. Keep a clear log of readings over several days.

Diagnosing High Blood Pressure

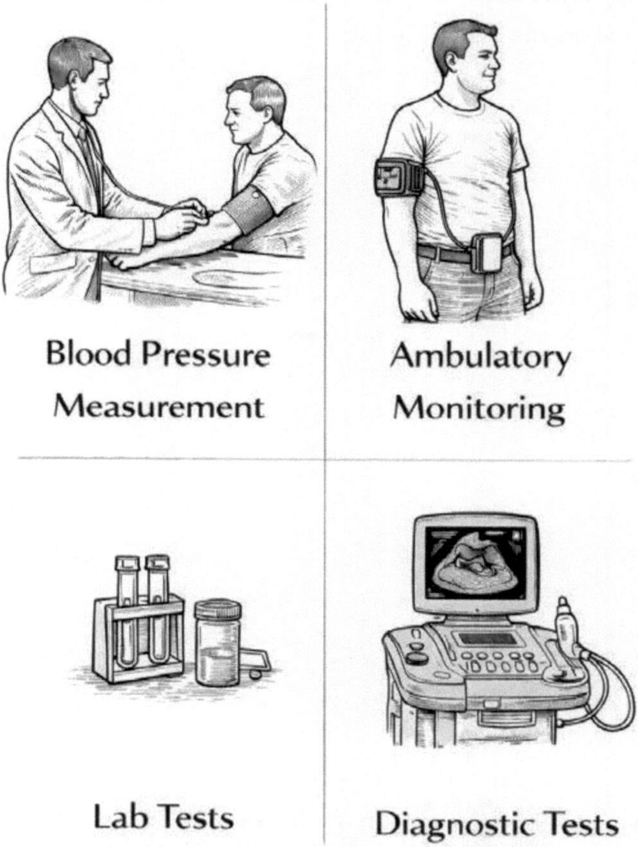

5. Share patterns with your clinician before starting or changing treatment.

Transition to Chapter 5

In the next chapter, we will connect blood pressure numbers to the real, long-term effects they can have on the heart, brain, kidneys, and other vital organs.

Chapter 5
The Damage High Blood Pressure Can Cause

High blood pressure is dangerous not because of how it feels today, but because of what it does quietly over time. Most people with elevated blood pressure feel normal for years. They go about daily life without discomfort or warning. Inside the body, however, persistent high pressure slowly strains delicate organs and blood vessels.

This is what makes high blood pressure especially harmful. It does not demand attention with pain or sudden symptoms. Instead, it causes gradual, silent injury. Understanding this connection between pressure and damage explains why treatment matters even when a person feels well.

This chapter explains how long-standing high blood pressure affects major organs and why early and steady control protects long-term health.

How High Blood Pressure Causes Damage

Blood vessels are designed to handle normal pressure comfortably. When pressure stays high for long periods, the inner lining of the vessels becomes injured. In response, vessel walls thicken and lose flexibility.

As arteries become stiffer and narrower, resistance to blood flow increases. The heart must pump harder to push blood through these vessels. This increased workload affects multiple organs over time.

Damage develops gradually. The body adapts and compensates for years before symptoms appear. By the time problems are noticed, significant injury may already be present. This is why prevention and early control are so important.

Effects on the Heart

The heart is often the first organ affected by long-term high blood pressure. Elevated pressure makes it harder for the heart to push blood into the arteries.

In response, the heart muscle thickens, especially on the left side. At first, this allows the heart to generate more force. Over time, however, the thickened muscle becomes stiff. A stiff heart does not relax or fill easily between beats.

This can lead to:

- Shortness of breath
- Reduced exercise tolerance
- Fluid buildup

- Irregular heart rhythms

Persistent strain also increases the risk of heart attack and heart failure. Lowering blood pressure reduces this strain and allows the heart to function more efficiently.

Effects on the Brain

The brain depends on a steady and well-regulated blood supply. High blood pressure disrupts this balance and is one of the strongest risk factors for stroke.

Constant pressure weakens blood vessel walls, increasing the risk of bleeding. At the same time, narrowed and damaged vessels are more likely to become blocked, cutting off blood flow to part of the brain.

High blood pressure also damages very small blood vessels in the brain. Over time, this can affect memory, concentration, and thinking speed. These changes are often mistaken for normal aging, but blood pressure plays a major role.

Protecting the brain is one of the strongest reasons to control blood pressure early and consistently.

Effects on the Kidneys

The kidneys help regulate blood pressure by controlling salt and fluid balance. They contain thousands of tiny blood vessels that filter waste from the blood.

High blood pressure damages these small vessels. As kidney function declines, the body becomes less efficient at removing salt and fluid. This raises blood pressure further and accelerates kidney damage.

This creates a harmful cycle. High blood pressure injures the kidneys. Injured kidneys raise blood pressure even more.

Kidney damage often develops silently. Blood tests may remain normal until significant injury has occurred. Early blood pressure control is one of the most effective ways to protect kidney function.

Effects on Eyes and Blood Vessels

High blood pressure affects blood vessels throughout the body, including those in the eyes.

Damage to the small vessels in the eyes can lead to vision changes and, in severe cases, permanent visual loss. Eye examinations can sometimes reveal blood pressure damage before symptoms appear elsewhere.

Blood vessels in other parts of the body may also narrow. Reduced circulation can cause discomfort during activity and delay healing.

Healthy blood vessels are essential for healthy organs. High blood pressure gradually compromises this system.

Why Long-Term Control Matters

Damage from high blood pressure does not happen all at once. It accumulates slowly over years.

The encouraging truth is that lowering blood pressure at any stage reduces risk. Even modest improvements can slow or stop further damage. Consistent control protects multiple organs at the same time.

The goal is not perfection, but stability. Keeping blood pressure within a safer range most of the time provides the greatest protection.

Two Everyday Examples

Example one:

A man avoids treatment because he feels well. Over time, his heart becomes enlarged and less efficient. Earlier control could have reduced this risk.

Example two:

A woman takes her diagnosis seriously and follows a steady treatment plan. Years later, her heart and kidney function remain strong. Early action made the difference.

Summary

- High blood pressure causes slow, silent damage
- Blood vessels become stiff and narrowed over time
- The heart works harder and may become stiff
- Stroke risk increases as brain vessels weaken
- Kidney damage develops quietly and worsens pressure
- Early and steady control reduces long-term harm

Steps for Getting an Accurate Blood Pressure Reading

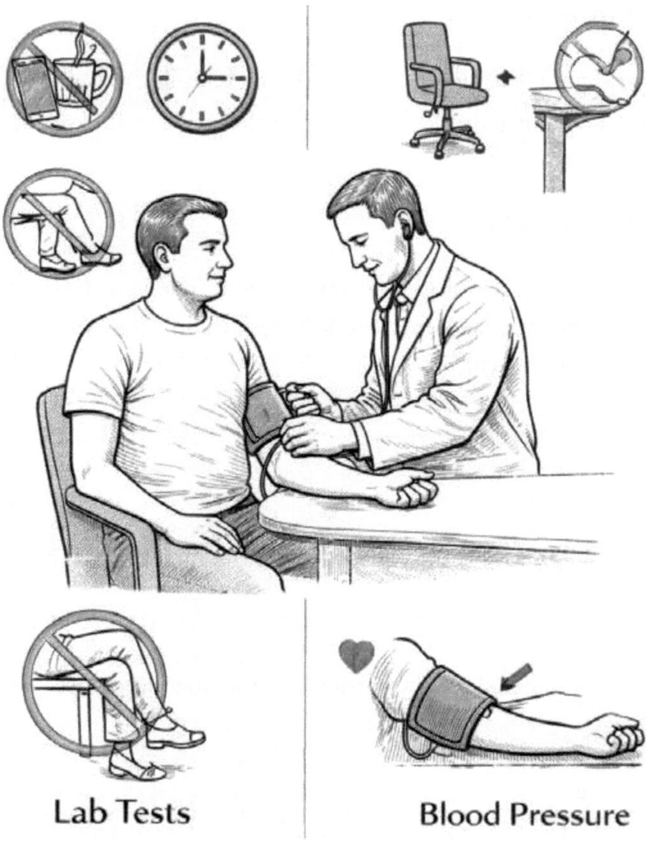

Your Practical Action Plan

1. Think beyond how you feel today and focus on long-term protection.
2. Take blood pressure treatment seriously even when you feel well.
3. Aim for steady control rather than occasional perfect readings.
4. Keep regular follow-up to detect early changes.
5. Remember that prevention is always easier than repair.

Transition to Chapter 6

In the next chapter, we will explore how everyday food choices influence blood pressure and how small, steady dietary changes can lead to meaningful improvement.

Chapter 6
Food, Salt, and Blood Pressure

Food influences blood pressure every single day. Unlike age or genetics, diet is a factor that can be adjusted at any stage of life. Many people are surprised to learn that small, consistent dietary changes often lower blood pressure as effectively as medication, especially in early stages.

This chapter explains how food affects blood pressure, why salt plays such a powerful role, and how everyday eating habits quietly shape blood pressure over time. The goal is not restriction or fear, but understanding. When people understand how food interacts with the body, better choices become easier and more sustainable.

How Food Affects Blood Pressure

Blood pressure responds to food in two main ways. First, certain foods influence how much salt and water the body retains. Second, food choices affect blood vessel health and flexibility.

When the body holds excess salt, it holds water along with it. This increases blood volume and raises pressure inside the arteries. At the same time, diets high in processed foods promote inflammation and stiffness in blood vessel walls, increasing resistance to blood flow.

In contrast, diets rich in fruits, vegetables, whole grains, and natural foods support flexible blood vessels and healthier circulation. These effects accumulate slowly, just as harmful effects do.

Understanding Salt Sensitivity

Not everyone responds to salt in the same way. Some people are salt sensitive, meaning their blood pressure rises significantly with higher sodium intake.

Salt sensitivity becomes more common with:

- Increasing age
- Family history of hypertension
- Kidney disease
- Diabetes
- Excess body weight

For salt-sensitive individuals, even modest reductions in sodium can produce meaningful blood pressure improvements. Others may see smaller changes, but still benefit from overall healthier eating.

Because it is impossible to know who is salt sensitive without reducing intake, moderation benefits almost everyone.

Hidden Sources of Sodium

Most dietary sodium does not come from salt added at the table. It comes from processed and prepared foods.

Common hidden sources include:

- Packaged snacks and frozen meals
- Restaurant foods
- Breads and baked goods
- Sauces, dressings, and condiments
- Processed meats

Even foods that do not taste salty may contain significant sodium. Reading labels and becoming aware of these sources is more effective than simply avoiding the saltshaker.

Gradual reduction allows taste buds to adjust. Over time, foods with excessive salt begin to taste unpleasant.

Healthy Eating Patterns That Lower Blood Pressure

Rather than focusing on individual foods, it is more helpful to focus on overall eating patterns.

Eating patterns that support healthy blood pressure share common features:

- Emphasis on fruits and vegetables
- Adequate intake of potassium-rich foods
- Preference for whole grains over refined grains
- Lean sources of protein

- Limited processed and packaged foods

These patterns improve blood vessel function, reduce inflammation, and support better weight management. They also benefit cholesterol levels, blood sugar, and overall cardiovascular health.

Food should support health, not create anxiety. Flexibility and balance are essential for long-term success.

Weight, Calories, and Blood Pressure

Excess body weight raises blood pressure through multiple mechanisms. A larger body requires more blood flow, increasing heart workload. Fat tissue also alters hormone signals that influence vessel tone and salt handling.

Even modest weight reduction can lower blood pressure. The goal is not rapid weight loss, but gradual and sustainable change.

Focusing on food quality often leads to natural calorie reduction without strict counting. This approach is more comfortable and easier to maintain over time.

Two Everyday Examples

Example one:

A man relies heavily on packaged foods due to a busy schedule. After reducing processed foods and cooking simple meals at home, his blood pressure improves. Awareness made the difference.

Example two:

A woman gradually lowers sodium intake and increases fruits and

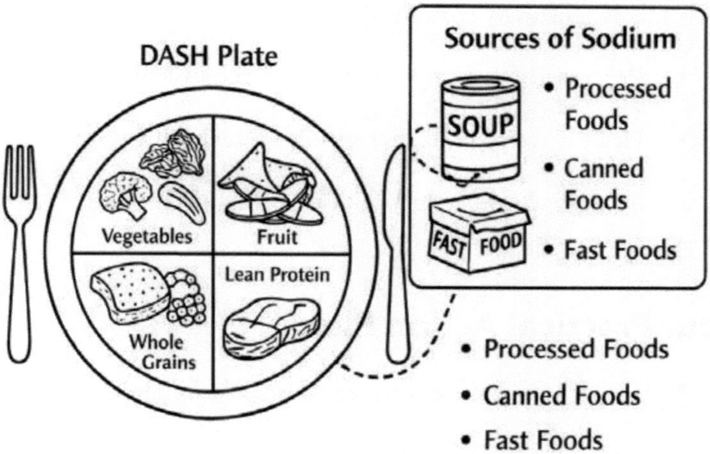

Lowering Blood Pressure *with* Food

vegetables. Over several months, her readings decline steadily without feeling deprived. Consistency mattered more than perfection.

Summary

- Food influences blood pressure daily
- Excess salt increases fluid retention and pressure
- Salt sensitivity varies but moderation benefits most people
- Processed foods are the main source of sodium
- Healthy eating patterns support vessel health
- Modest weight reduction lowers blood pressure

Your Practical Action Plan

1. Identify your main sources of dietary sodium.
2. Reduce processed and packaged foods gradually.
3. Increase fruits and vegetables at most meals.
4. Focus on eating patterns rather than strict rules.
5. Aim for steady, sustainable changes.

Transition to Chapter 7

In the next chapter, we will look beyond food and focus on lifestyle habits such as physical activity, sleep, and stress management, and how they influence blood pressure every day.

Chapter 7
Lifestyle Habits That Shape Blood Pressure

Blood pressure is influenced not only by food, but by how the body moves, rests, and responds to daily stress. These lifestyle factors work quietly in the background, shaping blood pressure from day to day. Many people focus on medication alone and underestimate how powerful daily habits can be.

Lifestyle changes do not need to be extreme to be effective. In fact, moderate and consistent habits often produce the most reliable results. This chapter explains how physical activity, sleep, stress, alcohol, and smoking influence blood pressure and how realistic changes can support long-term control.

Physical Activity and Blood Pressure

Regular physical activity lowers blood pressure in several important ways. Movement improves blood vessel flexibility, helps the body use insulin more efficiently, and reduces stress hormone levels.

When muscles work regularly, blood vessels become more responsive and relaxed. This lowers resistance to blood flow and reduces resting blood pressure. Physical activity also supports weight control, which further reduces pressure on the heart.

The goal is not intense exercise. Brisk walking, cycling, swimming, or similar activities performed most days of the week are enough to provide benefit. Consistency matters more than intensity.

Sedentary Behavior and Daily Movement

Long periods of sitting raise blood pressure independent of exercise. Even people who exercise regularly can see higher readings if most of the day is spent sitting.

Breaking up sitting time with brief movement improves circulation and reduces stiffness in blood vessels. Standing, stretching, or walking for a few minutes every hour supports healthier blood pressure patterns.

Daily movement is not separate from exercise. It is part of how the body stays balanced throughout the day.

Sleep and Blood Pressure Regulation

Healthy sleep allows blood pressure to fall naturally during the night. This nighttime drop gives blood vessels and the heart time to recover.

Poor or insufficient sleep disrupts this process. Blood pressure remains higher than it should be, even at rest. Over time, this contributes to sustained hypertension.

Conditions such as sleep apnea are especially important. Repeated interruptions in breathing activate stress responses and raise blood pressure both at night and during the day.

Protecting sleep quality and duration is a critical but often overlooked part of blood pressure care.

Stress and Emotional Health

Short-term stress causes temporary rises in blood pressure. This is normal. Problems arise when stress becomes constant.

Chronic stress keeps the body in a heightened state of alert. Stress hormones remain elevated, tightening blood vessels and increasing heart rate. Blood pressure begins to run higher even during periods of rest.

Managing stress does not require eliminating it. Simple practices such as structured routines, regular physical activity, relaxation techniques, and social connection can reduce its impact on blood pressure.

Alcohol, Tobacco, and Blood Pressure

Alcohol raises blood pressure in a dose-dependent way. Small amounts may have little effect, but regular or excessive intake raises readings and interferes with medications.

Smoking damages blood vessel lining and causes immediate tightening of arteries. While the blood pressure spike from smoking may be temporary, repeated exposure accelerates long-term vessel damage.

Reducing alcohol intake and avoiding tobacco are among the most powerful lifestyle steps for protecting blood vessels.

Two Everyday Examples

Example one:

A man adds daily walking and improves sleep consistency. Over several months, his blood pressure declines without additional medication. Small changes worked together.

Example two:

A woman experiences rising blood pressure during a stressful work period. By adjusting routines and reducing alcohol intake, her readings stabilize. Awareness made the difference.

Summary

- Physical activity improves vessel flexibility and lowers pressure
- Prolonged sitting raises blood pressure
- Healthy sleep allows nighttime pressure recovery
- Chronic stress keeps blood pressure elevated
- Alcohol and tobacco damage blood vessels
- Consistent habits support long-term control

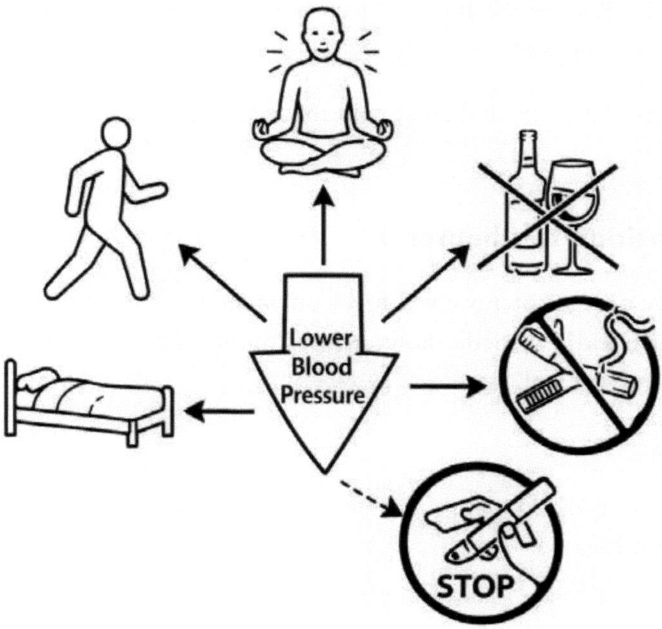

Exercise and *Lifestyle* Changes *That Really*

Your Practical Action Plan

1. Engage in moderate physical activity most days of the week.
2. Break up long periods of sitting with brief movement.
3. Protect sleep duration and consistency.
4. Reduce the impact of chronic stress through routine and support.
5. Limit alcohol and avoid tobacco.

Transition to Chapter 8

In the next chapter, we will focus on when lifestyle changes are not enough and how medications are used thoughtfully to support blood pressure control.

Chapter 8

Medicines Are Needed, When Lifestyle Changes Are Not Enough

Lifestyle changes form the foundation of blood pressure control. For many people, these steps are enough to keep readings in a healthy range. For others, however, blood pressure remains elevated despite sincere and consistent efforts. When this happens, it does not mean failure. It means the body needs additional support.

Blood pressure is influenced by genetics, age, vessel stiffness, and internal hormone systems. In some individuals, these forces are strong enough that lifestyle measures alone cannot fully overcome them. Medication is then used not as a substitute for healthy habits, but as a partner to them.

This chapter explains when medications are needed, why they are prescribed, and how they are used thoughtfully and safely.

Why Medication Becomes Necessary

Blood pressure remains high when the body's regulatory systems resist lifestyle adjustments. Arteries may stay narrowed. Kidneys may retain salt too efficiently. Stress hormone systems may remain overactive.

In these situations, medication helps reset balance. It reduces vessel resistance, lowers fluid volume, or calms hormonal signals. This allows blood pressure to move into a safer range and reduces ongoing strain on vital organs.

Medication is often recommended when:

- Blood pressure remains above target despite lifestyle efforts
- Overall cardiovascular risk is high
- Evidence of organ strain is present

The decision is based on protection, not urgency or fear.

Common Concerns About Starting Medication

Many people hesitate when medication is first discussed. Common worries include becoming dependent on pills, experiencing side effects, or needing treatment forever.

It is important to understand that blood pressure medication does not weaken the body. It supports systems that are under strain. Some people are able to reduce or stop medication later if circumstances change. Others need long-term treatment because the underlying tendencies persist.

Side effects are possible with any medication, but most blood pressure drugs are well tolerated, especially when started at low doses and adjusted gradually.

Open communication allows concerns to be addressed early and effectively.

How Doctors Choose Blood Pressure Medications

Medication selection is individualized. Doctors consider age, other medical conditions, kidney function, heart health, and potential interactions.

Different medications act on different systems. Some reduce fluid retention. Others relax blood vessels or slow heart workload. Often, low doses of two medications work better and cause fewer side effects than a high dose of one.

The goal is to lower blood pressure steadily without disrupting daily life.

Monitoring and Adjusting Treatment

Blood pressure treatment is rarely static. It evolves over time.

After starting medication, doctors monitor:

- Blood pressure response
- Symptoms or side effects
- Laboratory values when needed

Adjustments are common and expected. Dose changes, timing changes, or medication substitutions may be made to achieve better control with greater comfort.

Patients play a central role by reporting how they feel and sharing home blood pressure readings.

Medication and Lifestyle Work Together

Medication works best when combined with healthy habits. Lifestyle changes enhance medication effectiveness and may reduce the amount needed.

This partnership approach provides the greatest long-term protection. Medication lowers pressure while lifestyle habits support vessel health, weight control, and metabolic balance.

Viewing medication as a tool rather than a failure helps reduce resistance and improve adherence.

Two Everyday Examples

Example one:

A man follows lifestyle advice carefully, but his blood pressure remains high due to strong family history. Low-dose medication brings readings into range and protects his heart.

Example two:

A woman starts medication reluctantly but notices improved energy once blood pressure stabilizes. Combined with healthy habits, she maintains control comfortably.

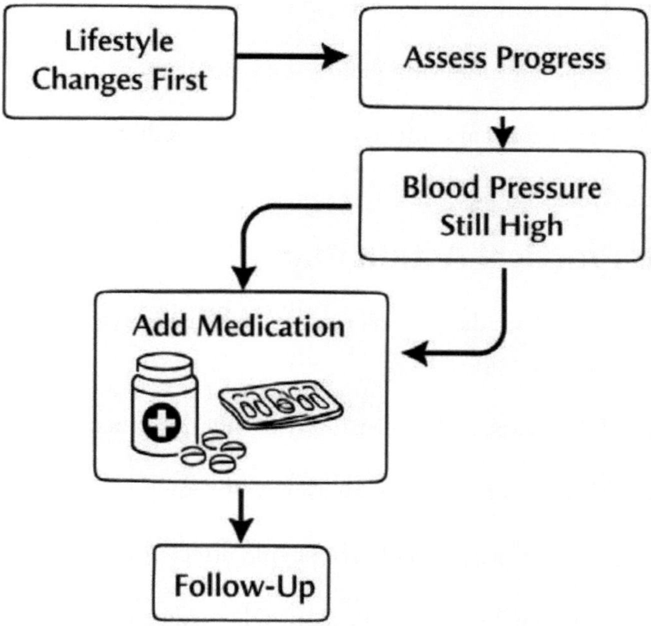

When Lifestyle *Changes Are Not Enough*

Summary

- Lifestyle changes are foundational but not always sufficient
- Medication supports internal systems that resist change
- Needing medication does not represent failure
- Treatment decisions are individualized
- Ongoing monitoring allows safe adjustment
- Medication and lifestyle work best together

Your Practical Action Plan

1. Accept medication as support when lifestyle changes are not enough.
2. Take medication consistently at the prescribed time.
3. Monitor blood pressure and symptoms regularly.
4. Communicate openly about side effects or concerns.
5. Continue healthy habits alongside medication.

Transition to Chapter 9

In the next chapter, we will explain the major blood pressure medication classes clearly, so you can understand what you are taking and why.

Chapter 9

Blood Pressure Medications Explained Clearly

By the time medication is prescribed, many people have the same questions. What does this medicine do? Why was this one chosen? Will I need it forever? These concerns are natural and deserve clear answers.

Blood pressure medications are not experimental or mysterious. Most have been used for decades and studied in millions of people. Each group works on a specific pressure-raising system in the body. Understanding these systems reduces fear and improves confidence.

This chapter explains the major blood pressure medication classes in plain language and shows how they protect the heart, brain, kidneys, and blood vessels over time.

Why There Are Different Medication Classes

Blood pressure rises through more than one pathway. Some people retain excess salt and water. Others have blood vessels that remain too tight. In some, the heart works harder than necessary. Because these mechanisms differ, treatment must be individualized.

Medication classes target different pathways:

- Fluid balance
- Blood vessel tone and elasticity
- Hormonal signals
- Heart workload

Choosing a medication is not guesswork. It is based on how a person's body behaves and what needs the most support.

Diuretics

Diuretics help the kidneys remove excess salt and water. When fluid volume decreases, pressure inside the arteries falls.

These medications are often used early because they are effective, affordable, and well studied. In low doses, they control blood pressure in many people.

Increased urination may occur at first, especially during the early weeks. This effect usually lessens as the body adjusts. Periodic blood tests may be used to ensure electrolyte balance.

A simple way to understand diuretics is to imagine releasing excess fluid from an overfilled system. Less volume means less pressure.

ACE Inhibitors and ARBs

ACE inhibitors and ARBs work on a hormone system that influences blood vessel tightening and salt balance. These medications relax blood vessels and reduce strain on the heart.

They are especially beneficial for people with diabetes, kidney disease, or heart disease because they offer protective effects beyond blood pressure lowering.

Some people develop a dry cough with ACE inhibitors. When this occurs, switching to an ARB usually resolves the problem while preserving benefits.

These medications are commonly used because of their effectiveness and long-term safety.

Calcium Channel Blockers

Calcium channel blockers reduce the movement of calcium into muscle cells in blood vessel walls. With less calcium, vessels relax and widen.

These medications are particularly helpful when arteries have become stiffer with age. Some people may notice ankle swelling or flushing, which can often be managed by adjusting the dose or timing.

By improving vessel relaxation, calcium channel blockers reduce resistance and lower blood pressure smoothly.

Beta Blockers and Other Agents

Beta blockers reduce heart rate and the force of contraction. This lowers the pressure generated with each heartbeat.

They are especially useful when high blood pressure is combined with heart rhythm problems, prior heart attack, or certain heart conditions. Not everyone with hypertension needs a beta blocker, but for some, they provide important protection.

Other medications may be used in special situations when additional control is needed. These choices are guided by individual response and tolerance.

Side Effects and Long-Term Safety

Most people tolerate blood pressure medications well. Side effects, when they occur, are usually mild and dose related.

Common effects include:

- Lightheadedness during early treatment
- Mild fatigue
- Ankle swelling with some medications

Starting with low doses and adjusting gradually reduces problems. Open communication allows timely adjustments before discomfort becomes a barrier.

Long-term studies consistently show that controlling blood pressure reduces heart attacks, strokes, and kidney disease.

Two Everyday Examples

Example one:

A man takes a diuretic and an ACE inhibitor. His blood pressure improves without side effects, and his kidney function remains stable. Understanding his medications improves confidence.

Example two:

A woman experiences ankle swelling on one medication. Her doctor adjusts treatment, and control is maintained comfortably. Flexibility leads to success.

Summary

- Blood pressure medications target different pressure-raising systems
- Multiple classes exist because causes vary
- Diuretics reduce fluid volume
- ACE inhibitors and ARBs relax vessels and protect organs
- Calcium channel blockers improve vessel flexibility
- Side effects are usually manageable

Your Practical Action Plan

1. Learn the names and purpose of your medications.
2. Take medications consistently at the same time each day.

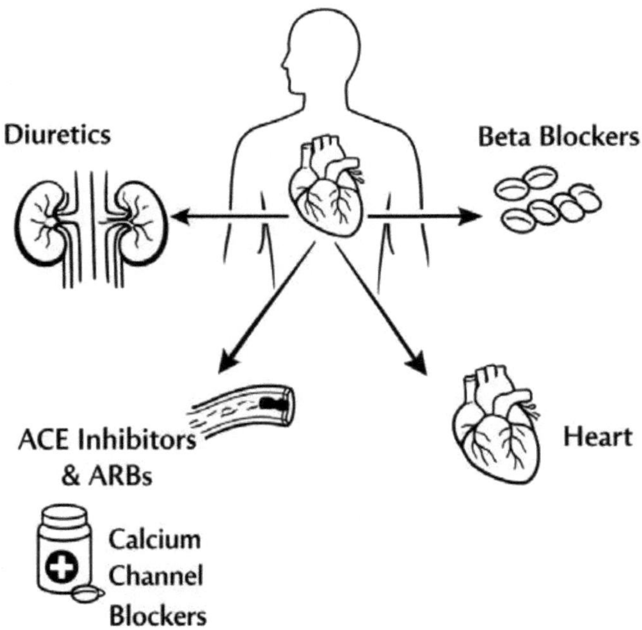

Blood Pressure Medications Explained *Clearly*

3. Monitor blood pressure and how you feel.
4. Report side effects early rather than stopping treatment.
5. View medication as protection, not punishment.

Transition to Chapter 10

In the next chapter, we will address special situations and difficult-to-control blood pressure, and explain how treatment is adapted when standard approaches are not enough.

Chapter 10

Special Situations and Difficult-to-Control Blood Pressure

High blood pressure does not behave the same way in every person. Some individuals respond quickly to lifestyle changes or a single medication. Others struggle despite careful treatment. When blood pressure proves difficult to control, it usually reflects additional influences rather than poor effort or failure.

Difficult-to-control blood pressure requires patience and careful evaluation. Understanding why control is challenging allows treatment to be adjusted safely and effectively. This chapter explains common special situations and how doctors approach blood pressure that does not respond as expected.

High Blood Pressure in Older Adults

With aging, blood vessels gradually lose flexibility. Healthy arteries expand with each heartbeat, absorbing pressure. Stiffer arteries resist this expansion, causing systolic pressure to rise while diastolic pressure may remain normal or even fall.

This pattern requires careful balance. Lowering systolic pressure protects the heart and brain, but overly aggressive treatment can cause dizziness, weakness, or falls.

In older adults, doctors focus on:

- Gradual dose adjustments
- Monitoring standing and seated blood pressure
- Watching for symptoms such as lightheadedness
- Preserving overall function and independence

Treatment aims for safety and stability rather than rapid change.

High Blood Pressure with Diabetes or Kidney Disease

Diabetes and kidney disease frequently coexist with high blood pressure. Each condition influences the others.

Diabetes damages small blood vessels, making blood pressure harder to control. Kidney disease interferes with salt and fluid regulation, often raising pressure further. Poor blood pressure control accelerates damage to both organs.

In these situations, blood pressure targets may be more specific. Certain medications offer added protection to the kidneys and heart beyond lowering numbers alone.

Careful monitoring and steady control slow disease progression and reduce complications.

Resistant Hypertension

Resistant hypertension refers to blood pressure that remains above target despite appropriate treatment with multiple medications, including a diuretic.

This situation is more common than many realize. It often reflects correctable factors rather than true treatment failure.

Common contributors include:

- High sodium intake
- Inconsistent medication use
- Inadequate medication combinations
- Unrecognized secondary causes

Addressing these issues frequently improves control. Resistant hypertension calls for careful review, not frustration.

Blood Pressure During Stress or Illness

Temporary elevations in blood pressure are common during illness, pain, emotional stress, or poor sleep. These rises reflect normal stress responses and usually settle once the underlying issue resolves.

Overreacting to short-term spikes can lead to unnecessary medication changes. Treatment decisions should be based on trends after recovery.

Understanding this pattern helps reduce anxiety and supports more thoughtful care.

When Specialist Care Is Helpful

Most people with high blood pressure are managed successfully in primary care. Specialist involvement may be helpful when blood pressure remains uncontrolled or behaves unusually.

Referral may be appropriate when:

- Blood pressure remains high despite careful treatment
- Secondary causes are suspected
- Kidney function is declining
- Medication side effects limit options

Team-based care often simplifies complex cases and improves outcomes.

Two Everyday Examples

Example one:

A man takes several medications but continues high salt intake. After dietary review and adjustment, his blood pressure improves. Identifying contributors made the difference.

Example two:

A woman with kidney disease requires careful medication selection and close monitoring. Individualized treatment stabilizes her blood pressure safely.

Resistant Hypertension *Checklist*

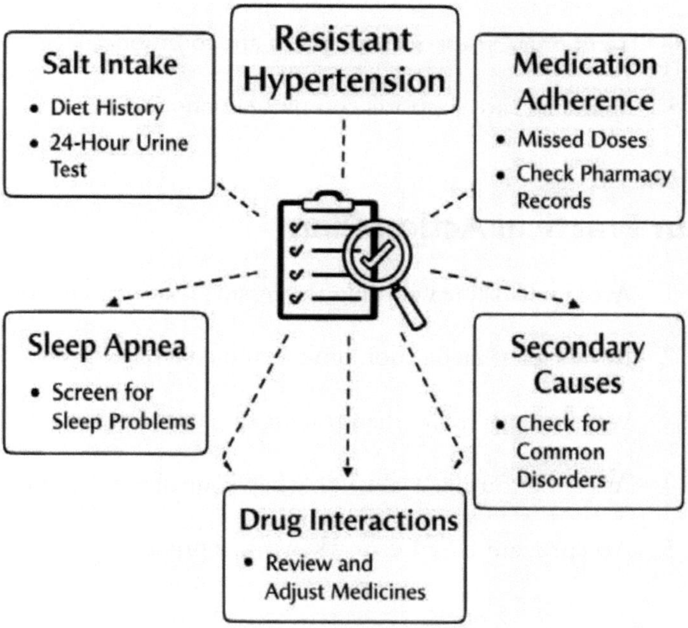

Summary

- Blood pressure control varies between individuals
- Aging affects vessel flexibility and treatment goals
- Diabetes and kidney disease complicate management
- Resistant hypertension often has correctable causes
- Temporary stress-related spikes are common
- Specialist care supports complex situations

Your Practical Action Plan

1. Avoid self-blame when blood pressure is difficult to control.
2. Review diet, medication timing, and adherence honestly.
3. Watch trends rather than reacting to isolated spikes.
4. Ask about further evaluation when control remains difficult.
5. Accept team-based care when appropriate.

Transition to Chapter 11

In the next chapter, we will bring everything together into a clear, practical plan for controlling blood pressure safely and confidently for life.

Chapter 11

Your Practical Plan to Control Blood Pressure for Life

Understanding blood pressure is important, but understanding alone does not protect health. What truly matters is how knowledge is translated into daily habits over months and years. This final chapter brings everything together into a practical, realistic approach that fits ordinary life.

Good blood pressure control is not achieved through intensity or short bursts of effort. It is built quietly, through small actions repeated consistently. People who succeed are not those who aim for perfection, but those who commit to steady care and flexibility.

This chapter focuses on turning understanding into long-term protection.

Setting Realistic Blood Pressure Goals

Blood pressure goals are not identical for everyone. Age, medical history, and overall cardiovascular risk influence what is appropriate.

Rather than chasing perfect numbers, the focus should be on maintaining blood pressure in a safer range most of the time. Occasional higher readings are normal and expected. Stress, illness, travel, or poor sleep can all cause temporary increases.

Progress should be judged by trends over weeks and months. A calm, long-term perspective prevents frustration and supports adherence.

Creating a Personal Blood Pressure Plan

A clear plan reduces uncertainty and improves confidence. When people know what they are working toward, decisions become easier.

An effective blood pressure plan usually includes:

- Thoughtful food choices with reduced sodium
- Regular physical activity
- Attention to sleep and stress
- Consistent medication use when needed
- Periodic monitoring and follow-up

The best plan fits naturally into daily routines. It should support life, not disrupt it. Plans that are overly strict often fail, while flexible plans tend to last.

Monitoring Without Anxiety

Monitoring blood pressure is meant to inform, not alarm. Used correctly, it provides clarity and reassurance.

Helpful monitoring habits include:

- Measuring at consistent times
- Using proper technique
- Recording readings accurately
- Sharing results with your clinician

Monitoring helps distinguish temporary changes from meaningful trends. It prevents overreaction and guides thoughtful adjustments.

Working in Partnership with Your Doctor

Blood pressure care works best as a partnership. Honest communication matters more than perfect behavior.

Sharing concerns, side effects, missed doses, or lifestyle challenges allows treatment to be adjusted realistically. Doctors can only help with what they know.

When patients and clinicians work together, treatment becomes simpler, safer, and more effective.

Staying Consistent Over Time

Motivation naturally rises and falls. Habits provide stability when motivation fades.

Simple strategies support consistency:

- Linking medication to daily routines
- Keeping goals visible
- Allowing setbacks without self-criticism
- Focusing on progress rather than perfection

Blood pressure control is not a test to pass or fail. It is an ongoing process that allows adjustment and learning.

Two Everyday Examples

Example one:

A woman develops a steady routine for meals, walking, and medication. Years later, her blood pressure remains controlled without stress. Consistency protected her health.

Example two:

A man experiences setbacks during a busy period. Instead of giving up, he revisits his plan and makes small corrections. Control returns gradually.

Summary

- Long-term control depends on steady habits
- Goals should be realistic and individualized
- Monitoring guides decisions without fear

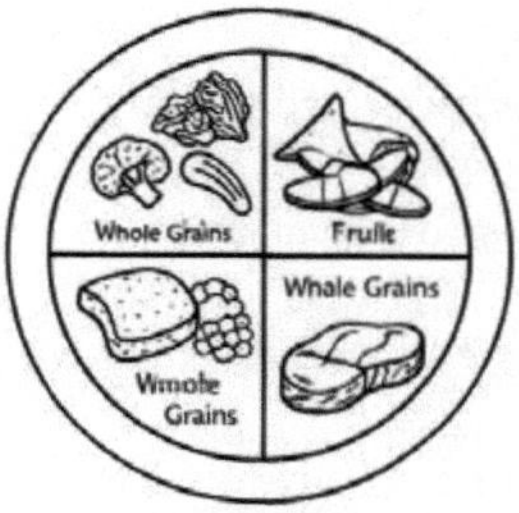

Healthy Diet

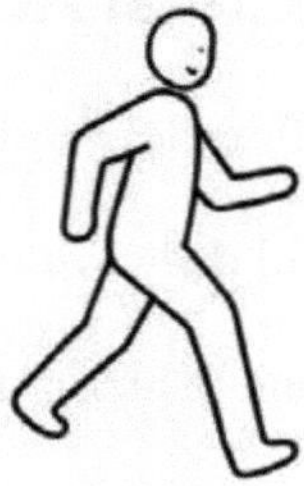

Exercise

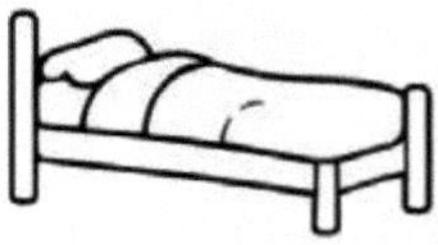

Good Sleep

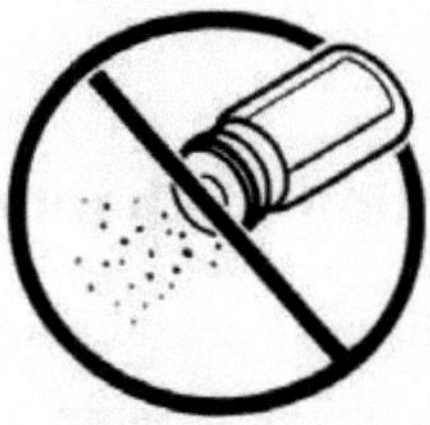

Limit Salt

How to Prevent High *Blood Pressure*

- Partnership with your doctor improves outcomes
- Consistency matters more than intensity
- Small actions repeated over time protect health

Your Practical Action Plan

1. Define clear and realistic blood pressure goals.
2. Build daily routines that support those goals.
3. Monitor blood pressure thoughtfully and consistently.
4. Communicate openly with your healthcare provider.
5. Stay patient and flexible over time.

Transition to Chapter 12

In the next chapter, we will explore myths and misconceptions related to high blood pressure.

Chapter 12

Common Myths and Misconceptions About High Blood Pressure

High blood pressure is surrounded by myths. These myths are not harmless. They delay diagnosis, weaken treatment, and create unnecessary fear or false reassurance. Over the years, I have seen many intelligent, well-meaning people make poor decisions simply because they believed something that sounded logical but was medically incorrect.

This chapter addresses the most common misconceptions about high blood pressure. Clearing these misunderstandings is just as important as explaining medications or lifestyle changes. When myths fall away, good decisions become easier and more consistent.

Myth 1: "I Feel Fine, So My Blood Pressure Must Be Fine"

This is the most dangerous myth of all.

High blood pressure is often called the silent condition for a reason. Most people feel completely normal, sometimes for decades. There is no pain, no warning signal, and no early symptom that reliably indicates rising pressure.

The body adapts quietly to higher pressure, even as damage slowly develops in the heart, brain, kidneys, and blood vessels. Feeling well does not mean blood pressure is normal. It only means symptoms have not yet appeared.

Blood pressure must be measured to be known. There is no other reliable way.

Myth 2: "Stress Is the Only Cause of High Blood Pressure"

Stress does raise blood pressure temporarily, and chronic stress can contribute to long-term elevation. However, stress is rarely the only cause.

Blood pressure is influenced by multiple factors working together:

- Age and genetics
- Salt sensitivity
- Weight and physical activity
- Sleep quality
- Hormonal regulation

Many people with calm personalities develop high blood pressure. Many highly stressed individuals do not. Stress is one piece of a larger picture.

Managing stress is helpful, but it is not a substitute for comprehensive care.

Myth 3: "Once My Blood Pressure Is Normal, I Can Stop Everything"

When blood pressure improves, people often assume the problem is gone. In reality, improvement usually reflects successful management, not cure.

Lifestyle changes and medications work by counteracting underlying tendencies. When those supports are removed, blood pressure often rises again.

In some cases, medication doses can be reduced or stopped under supervision, especially when weight loss, diet, and activity improve significantly. But this decision must be thoughtful and monitored.

Stopping treatment abruptly or on one's own is a common reason blood pressure becomes uncontrolled again.

Myth 4: "Blood Pressure Medicines Damage the Kidneys"

This myth causes unnecessary fear and medication avoidance.

In reality, uncontrolled high blood pressure is one of the leading causes of kidney damage. Many blood pressure medications actually protect kidney function, especially in people with diabetes or early kidney disease.

Doctors monitor kidney function and electrolytes when appropriate.

When problems arise, medications are adjusted. Serious kidney injury from properly prescribed blood pressure medication is uncommon.

The greater risk lies in leaving blood pressure untreated.

Myth 5: "Natural Remedies Are Enough"

Lifestyle changes are powerful. Diet, physical activity, weight control, and sleep can significantly lower blood pressure. In early or mild cases, they may be enough.

However, when blood pressure remains high despite these efforts, relying solely on natural approaches becomes risky. This does not mean lifestyle changes have failed. It means the body needs additional support.

Medication and lifestyle are not opposing approaches. They work best together. Rejecting one in favor of the other often leads to poorer outcomes.

Myth 6: "High Blood Pressure Is Just a Part of Getting Older"

Blood pressure tends to rise with age, but that does not mean it should be ignored.

Aging changes blood vessels, but treatment still reduces the risk of stroke, heart failure, and kidney disease. The goal in older adults is balance, not neglect.

Accepting high blood pressure as inevitable removes the opportunity for protection. Even modest control provides meaningful benefit at any age.

Myth 7: "One High Reading Means I Have Hypertension"

Blood pressure naturally fluctuates. A single high reading does not define a diagnosis.

Activity, stress, pain, caffeine, and anxiety can temporarily raise readings. Diagnosis is based on repeated measurements taken correctly over time.

At the same time, repeated high readings should not be dismissed. Both overreaction and underreaction cause harm. Thoughtful evaluation prevents both.

Two Everyday Examples

Example one:

A man avoids medication because he feels well and believes stress is the only cause. Years later, he develops heart strain that could have been prevented. The myth delayed protection.

Example two:

A woman fears medication will harm her kidneys. After learning that uncontrolled blood pressure poses the real risk, she accepts treatment and preserves kidney function. Correct information changed her path.

Summary

- High blood pressure is often symptom-free

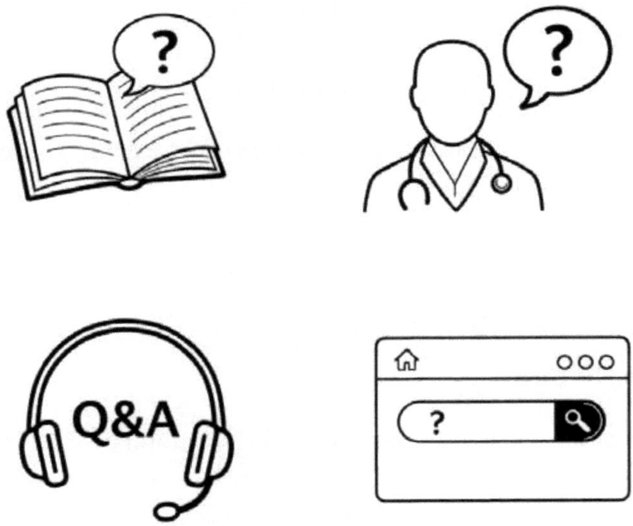

Answers to Common Questions

- Stress is rarely the only cause
- Improvement does not equal cure
- Blood pressure medicines protect organs
- Lifestyle and medication work together
- Aging does not eliminate the need for treatment
- Diagnosis requires patterns, not single readings

Your Practical Action Plan

1. Question beliefs that delay measurement or treatment.
2. Focus on long-term protection rather than short-term comfort.
3. Combine lifestyle changes with medication when needed.
4. Avoid stopping treatment without medical guidance.
5. Replace myths with reliable information.

Transition to Chapter 13

In the next chapter, we will explore how blood pressure changes across different stages of life and why treatment strategies evolve with age.

Chapter 13

Blood Pressure Across Different Stages of Life

Blood pressure is not static. It changes as the body changes. Age, hormones, vessel flexibility, metabolism, and life circumstances all influence how blood pressure behaves over time. Understanding these shifts reduces confusion and helps people accept why treatment plans may need adjustment at different stages of life.

Many patients ask a simple question. "Why is my blood pressure different now than it was ten or twenty years ago?" The answer lies in how the cardiovascular system adapts, and sometimes struggles to adapt, as we age.

This chapter explains how blood pressure typically behaves across adult life and why management strategies evolve with time.

Blood Pressure in Early Adulthood

In the twenties and thirties, blood vessels are usually flexible and resilient. The heart pumps efficiently, and regulatory systems respond quickly to stress or activity.

When high blood pressure appears at this stage, it often reflects strong genetic influence, obesity, high salt intake, sleep disruption, or secondary causes. Readings may fluctuate and normalize easily with lifestyle changes.

At this stage, the emphasis is on:

- Accurate diagnosis
- Lifestyle correction
- Identifying secondary causes when appropriate

Early intervention can delay or prevent long-term complications. This is a period when habits have lasting impact.

Blood Pressure in the Forties and Fifties

This is a common turning point. Many people first encounter consistently elevated blood pressure during these decades.

Several changes occur together:

- Gradual stiffening of arteries
- Weight gain around the abdomen
- Reduced physical activity
- Increasing work and life stress
- Subtle sleep disruption

Blood pressure may rise slowly and remain unnoticed for years unless measured regularly. Lifestyle changes remain powerful, but medications are often needed to maintain control.

This stage is critical because early treatment greatly reduces later heart, brain, and kidney damage.

Blood Pressure After Sixty

With advancing age, systolic pressure often rises while diastolic pressure stabilizes or falls. This reflects increasing arterial stiffness rather than overactive circulation.

Treatment priorities shift slightly. Lowering systolic pressure remains important, but care must be taken to avoid dizziness, falls, or weakness.

Doctors focus on:

- Gradual dose adjustments
- Monitoring standing blood pressure
- Preserving balance and independence
- Avoiding overly aggressive targets

Even at this stage, controlling blood pressure reduces stroke and heart failure risk. Age changes strategy, not purpose.

Differences Between Men and Women

Hormonal factors influence blood pressure patterns. Before menopause, women often have lower blood pressure than men. After menopause, this difference narrows or reverses.

Changes in estrogen levels affect vessel flexibility and salt handling. Weight distribution also shifts, influencing blood pressure.

Pregnancy-related conditions, such as gestational hypertension, increase long-term risk later in life. Awareness allows earlier monitoring and prevention.

Treatment principles remain the same, but timing and progression often differ.

Blood Pressure with Other Medical Conditions

As people age, additional conditions become more common. Diabetes, kidney disease, heart disease, and sleep apnea all interact with blood pressure.

These conditions may:

- Raise blood pressure
- Make control more difficult
- Change medication choices
- Influence treatment targets

In such cases, blood pressure management becomes part of a broader care plan rather than an isolated goal.

Why Treatment Plans Change Over Time

Many patients worry when medications are adjusted or added. They assume something has gone wrong.

In reality, change often reflects appropriate adaptation. The body evolves. Treatment must evolve with it.

A medication that worked well ten years ago may need adjustment today. This is not failure. It is good medicine.

Understanding this prevents frustration and improves long-term adherence.

Two Everyday Examples

Example one:

A man controls blood pressure with lifestyle changes in his forties. In his fifties, rising readings require medication. Early habits still reduce the amount needed.

Example two:

A woman develops higher systolic pressure after menopause. Treatment is adjusted gradually, protecting her health without causing dizziness. Care evolves with age.

Summary

- Blood pressure changes across adult life
- Early adulthood allows strong lifestyle impact
- Midlife often marks sustained elevation
- Aging increases arterial stiffness
- Men and women show different patterns

- Other conditions influence management
- Treatment adjustment reflects adaptation

Your Practical Action Plan

1. Measure blood pressure regularly as you age.
2. Accept that treatment needs may change over time.
3. Maintain healthy habits at every stage of life.
4. Report new symptoms or side effects promptly.
5. Focus on long-term protection rather than past comparisons.

Transition to Chapter 14

In the next chapter, we will address the most common questions patients ask about high blood pressure, medications, monitoring, and daily life, bringing clarity to concerns that arise in real-world practice.

Chapter 14

Frequently Asked Questions Patients Ask Their Doctor

After understanding blood pressure, its causes, and its treatment, many practical questions remain. These are the questions patients ask quietly in the exam room, or think about later at home. They are not signs of doubt or weakness. They are signs of engagement and responsibility.

This chapter addresses the most common questions I hear in everyday practice. Clear answers reduce anxiety, improve adherence, and help people feel confident rather than overwhelmed.

"Will I Need Blood Pressure Medicine for the Rest of My Life?"

Not necessarily, but sometimes yes.

Blood pressure medication is prescribed to counteract forces that are raising pressure. If those forces change, medication needs may change as well. Weight loss, improved diet, better sleep, and regular physical activity can sometimes reduce or eliminate the need for medication.

However, if blood pressure remains high due to age, genetics, or vessel stiffness, long-term medication may be the safest option. Taking medication long term is not a failure. It is a form of protection.

The goal is not to avoid medication at all costs, but to protect the heart, brain, and kidneys effectively.

"What Happens If I Miss a Dose?"

Missing an occasional dose happens to almost everyone. One missed dose usually does not cause harm, but repeated missed doses can allow blood pressure to rise again.

If you remember within a few hours, take the dose unless advised otherwise. If it is close to the next scheduled dose, skip the missed one and resume your regular schedule. Do not double doses unless instructed.

If missed doses are frequent, the solution is not guilt. It is adjusting routines to make adherence easier.

"Why Are My Home Readings Different from Office Readings?"

This is very common and often expected.

Home readings are taken in a familiar, relaxed environment. Office readings may be influenced by anxiety, time pressure, or conversation.

Both are useful, but they measure slightly different situations.

What matters most is:

- Correct technique
- Consistency
- Trends over time

Doctors often rely more on home readings to guide treatment, especially when office readings are borderline or inconsistent.

"How Often Should I Check My Blood Pressure?"

Frequency depends on the situation.

When blood pressure is newly diagnosed or treatment is being adjusted, checking once or twice daily for a few days each week is reasonable. Once control is stable, less frequent monitoring is often sufficient.

Checking too often can increase anxiety without improving outcomes. Monitoring should inform decisions, not dominate daily life.

"Can Blood Pressure Medicine Be Stopped Suddenly?"

Most blood pressure medications should not be stopped abruptly. Sudden withdrawal can cause blood pressure to rise quickly and, in some cases, lead to serious complications.

Any decision to stop or reduce medication should be made gradually and under medical supervision. If side effects occur, adjustment is safer than sudden discontinuation.

"Are Blood Pressure Medications Addictive?"

No.

Blood pressure medications do not cause dependence or craving. The body does not become addicted to them. The need for ongoing treatment reflects underlying physiology, not addiction.

This distinction is important. Taking medication because it is beneficial is not the same as being dependent on it.

"Can I Drink Alcohol While Taking Blood Pressure Medication?"

Alcohol can raise blood pressure and interfere with medication effectiveness. Small amounts may be acceptable for some people, but regular or excessive intake raises risk.

Alcohol also increases dizziness and lightheadedness when combined with certain medications. Moderation is key, and discussion with your doctor helps clarify what is safe for you.

"Why Does My Doctor Keep Adjusting My Medications?"

Adjustment does not mean something is wrong. It means treatment is being tailored.

Blood pressure changes with age, weight, stress, sleep, and other medical conditions. Medication adjustment reflects careful attention, not uncertainty.

Good treatment evolves as the body evolves.

Two Everyday Examples

Example one:

A man becomes anxious because his home readings differ from office readings. After reviewing proper technique and trends, unnecessary medication changes are avoided. Understanding reduced worry.

Example two:

A woman misses doses during travel and sees higher readings. By linking medication to daily routines, control improves. Small adjustments restored stability.

Summary

- Many blood pressure concerns are common and reasonable
- Medication duration varies by individual
- Occasional missed doses are manageable
- Home readings often guide treatment
- Sudden medication changes can be risky
- Adjustment reflects good care, not failure

Your Practical Action Plan

1. Ask questions whenever something feels unclear.
2. Use home blood pressure readings thoughtfully.
3. Take medications consistently and safely.
4. Avoid abrupt changes without guidance.
5. Focus on understanding rather than fear.

Chapter 15

Why Many People Hesitate to Start Blood Pressure Medication

One of the most common conversations I have with patients does not begin with numbers or test results. It begins with hesitation. Many people understand that their blood pressure is high, yet feel strongly that they want to manage it without medication. This preference is understandable, and it deserves thoughtful discussion rather than dismissal.

Reluctance to start medication does not usually come from ignorance or stubbornness. It comes from fear, past experiences, misinformation, and a desire to remain in control of one's health. This chapter explores why so many people resist starting blood pressure medicine and how these concerns can be addressed calmly and rationally.

The Desire to Fix the Problem Naturally

Many people believe that if they try hard enough, lifestyle changes alone should be sufficient. Eating better, exercising more, losing weight, reducing stress, and sleeping well all feel like healthier and more dignified solutions than taking a daily pill.

This belief is not wrong. Lifestyle changes are powerful and form the foundation of blood pressure management. In early or mild hypertension, they may be enough. The difficulty arises when blood pressure remains elevated despite sincere effort.

The body does not always respond as we hope. Genetics, vessel stiffness, kidney function, and hormonal regulation may continue to push pressure higher even in the face of healthy habits. When this happens, medication becomes support rather than surrender.

Fear of Becoming Dependent on Medicine

A common worry is, "Once I start medicine, I will never be able to stop." This fear is deeply rooted and often reinforced by stories from friends or family.

Blood pressure medicines do not create dependence. They do not weaken the body's ability to regulate itself. They simply assist systems that are under strain. Some people are able to reduce or stop medication later when circumstances change. Others need long-term treatment because the underlying tendency persists.

Needing medication does not mean the body has failed. It means the body needs help.

Concern About Side Effects

Many patients worry about side effects before they ever take a pill. They imagine fatigue, dizziness, kidney damage, or long-term harm.

While side effects are possible with any medication, most blood pressure medicines are well tolerated. Doctors usually start with low doses and adjust gradually. Monitoring allows early detection of problems, and alternatives are available if one medication does not suit a person.

The greater risk comes from leaving blood pressure untreated. The silent damage caused by high pressure is far more dangerous than the side effects most people fear.

Influence of Misinformation

The internet and social media have changed how health information spreads. Unfortunately, misinformation spreads faster than balanced medical advice.

People often encounter claims that:

- Medication is unnecessary if lifestyle is perfect
- Natural supplements can replace proven treatments
- Doctors prescribe medication too quickly
- Medicines are promoted for profit rather than health

These messages are persuasive, especially when they promise control without compromise. What they often ignore is evidence, long-term outcomes, and individual variation.

Reliable medical advice does not dismiss lifestyle changes. It integrates them with treatments proven to reduce heart attacks, strokes, and kidney failure.

Feeling That Starting Medication Means Failure

For some people, starting medication feels like admitting defeat. They feel they should have done more, tried harder, or been more disciplined.

This emotional response is common and understandable, but it is misplaced. Blood pressure is influenced by many factors beyond personal effort. Accepting medication is not a judgment of character or willpower.

In reality, choosing appropriate treatment reflects responsibility, not failure. It shows a willingness to protect long-term health rather than cling to an idealized notion of control.

The Hope That Waiting Will Be Harmless

Because high blood pressure often causes no symptoms, many people believe they have time. They plan to delay medication and see what happens.

Unfortunately, damage does not wait for symptoms. Blood vessels, the heart, the brain, and the kidneys are affected quietly. Waiting without control increases long-term risk even when a person feels well.

Early control does not lock someone into permanent medication. It protects organs while decisions are made thoughtfully.

How Doctors View Non-Medication Management

Doctors strongly support non-medication strategies. Diet, physical activity, weight management, sleep, and stress reduction are essential parts of care.

When medication is recommended, it is not because lifestyle has failed. It is because lifestyle alone has not been enough to overcome the body's internal pressures.

Medication and lifestyle are not competing approaches. They are complementary. When used together, they offer the greatest protection.

Two Everyday Examples

Example one:

A man delays medication for years, hoping lifestyle alone will work. By the time he agrees to treatment, early heart changes are present. Earlier support could have reduced risk.

Example two:

A woman resists medication initially but agrees after understanding its role. Combined with lifestyle changes, her blood pressure stabilizes, and she later reduces her dose. Partnership made the difference.

Summary

- Many people prefer non-medication approaches
- Fear, misinformation, and emotion play major roles
- Lifestyle changes are essential but not always sufficient
- Blood pressure medicines do not cause dependence
- Side effects are usually manageable
- Delaying treatment carries silent risks
- Medication supports, rather than replaces, healthy habits

Your Practical Action Plan

1. Acknowledge concerns about medication without judgment.
2. Commit fully to lifestyle changes regardless of treatment choice.
3. Evaluate blood pressure response honestly over time.
4. Accept medication as support if targets are not reached.
5. Focus on long-term protection rather than short-term comfort.

Chapter 16

Taking Your Blood Pressure Correctly

Blood pressure numbers are only useful if they are accurate. Unfortunately, many readings taken at home, in pharmacies, or even in clinics are affected by small but important errors. These mistakes can lead to unnecessary worry, incorrect diagnosis, or inappropriate treatment changes.

In this chapter, I want to show you how to take your blood pressure correctly, explain the most common mistakes people make, and offer simple remedies to improve accuracy. When blood pressure is measured properly, it becomes a reliable guide rather than a source of confusion.

1) Why Correct Measurement Matters

Blood pressure changes from moment to moment. It rises with activity, stress, pain, and even conversation. A poorly taken reading can easily be higher than your true resting blood pressure.

An inaccurate reading may lead to:

Unnecessary anxiety

Incorrect diagnosis of hypertension

Overtreatment or undertreatment

Confusing or conflicting advice

When blood pressure is measured correctly and consistently, patterns become clear and decisions become safer.

2) Preparing for an Accurate Reading

Good measurement begins before the cuff is even applied.

To prepare properly:

Rest quietly for at least five minutes

Avoid exercise, smoking, or caffeine for thirty minutes before measuring

Empty your bladder

Sit in a calm, quiet environment

Rushing into a measurement immediately after activity almost always produces a falsely high reading.

Everyday example:

A person checks blood pressure immediately after climbing stairs. The reading is high. Ten minutes later, after resting, the numbers are much lower and more accurate.

3) Correct Body Position and Technique

Position matters more than most people realize.

Follow these steps carefully:

Sit upright with your back supported

Keep both feet flat on the floor

Do not cross your legs

Support your arm on a table

Keep the cuff at heart level

Relax and remain silent during measurement

The cuff should fit properly. A cuff that is too small can falsely raise readings, while a cuff that is too large can lower them.

If you are using a home monitor, upper-arm devices are generally more reliable than wrist or finger monitors.

4) Common Mistakes That Affect Readings

Many blood pressure errors are subtle and easy to overlook.

Common mistakes include:

Talking during measurement

Holding the arm in the air

Measuring over clothing

Sitting on the edge of a chair without back support

Crossing legs

Using the wrong cuff size

Taking readings immediately after stress or activity

Each of these can raise systolic blood pressure by several points. When combined, they can significantly distort results.

5) Home Blood Pressure Monitoring Tips

Home monitoring can be extremely helpful when done correctly.

Helpful guidelines include:

Measure at the same time each day

Take two readings, one minute apart

Record both numbers

Avoid checking too frequently

Checking too often can increase anxiety and lead to overinterpretation of normal fluctuations.

Everyday example:

A patient checks blood pressure once in the morning and once in the evening for a week. The average readings provide a clear and reliable picture.

6) Office, Pharmacy, and Ambulatory Measurements

Blood pressure measured in a clinic may be higher due to anxiety. This is sometimes called white-coat effect. On the other hand, some people have normal office readings but elevated pressures at home.

Ambulatory blood pressure monitoring, which measures blood pressure over twenty four hours, can provide valuable information in selected cases. It shows daytime and nighttime patterns and helps confirm diagnosis when readings are unclear.

No single reading tells the whole story. Patterns matter far more than isolated numbers.

Summary

Blood pressure readings are only meaningful when taken correctly.

Small errors can significantly affect results.

Proper preparation, posture, and cuff placement are essential.

Home monitoring is useful when done consistently and calmly.

Trends over time matter more than single readings.

Your Practical Action Plan

Create a quiet routine for blood pressure measurement.

Use the same chair, arm position, and time of day.

Avoid common mistakes such as talking or crossing legs.

Taking Your Blood Pressure Correctly

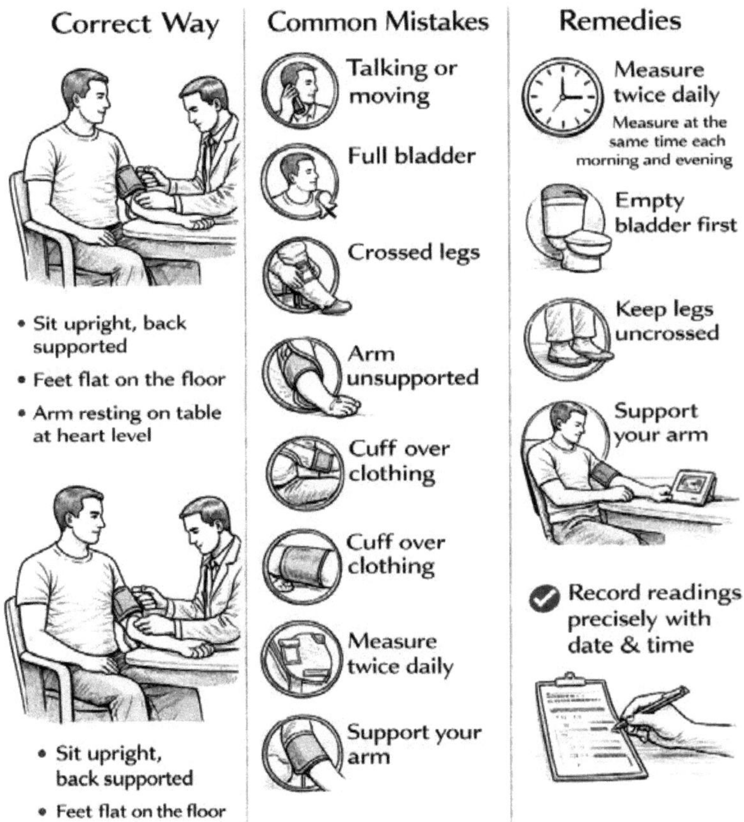

Record readings clearly and bring them to appointments.

Focus on averages, not occasional spikes.

Correct blood pressure measurement is a skill. Once learned, it gives you confidence, clarity, and control. When numbers are accurate, decisions become easier and care becomes safer.

Chapter 17

Conclusion: Final Message to the Reader

Thank you for spending your time with this book. Choosing to read and understand your health is, in itself, a meaningful step. It reflects responsibility, curiosity, and a desire to care for yourself and those who depend on you.

Managing blood pressure is not about mastering rules or chasing numbers. It is about understanding your body, working in partnership with your doctor, and making steady choices that protect health over time. When questions are answered clearly and decisions are made calmly, blood pressure becomes a manageable part of life rather than a constant source of worry.

High blood pressure often begins quietly and travels with us for years. For many people, it is discovered by chance during a routine visit, when life otherwise feels normal. That moment can bring confusion, worry, or even denial. This book was written to replace those feelings with understanding, clarity, and calm confidence.

Blood pressure is not an enemy. It is a signal. It reflects how the heart, blood vessels, kidneys, and nervous system are responding to daily life. When that signal stays high, it deserves attention, not fear. With knowledge and steady care, high blood pressure becomes manageable and predictable rather than threatening.

One of the most important messages to carry forward is this. Good blood pressure control is rarely about dramatic change. It is about small, sensible decisions repeated consistently. Choosing better food most days. Moving the body regularly. Sleeping well. Managing stress with intention. Taking medication thoughtfully when needed. None of these actions is extreme, but together they are powerful.

Another important lesson is patience. Blood pressure does not rise overnight, and it rarely improves overnight. Progress often appears gradually. Occasional setbacks are normal. What matters is returning to the plan without self-criticism. Long-term success belongs to those who stay engaged rather than those who seek perfection.

This book has emphasized partnership. Partnership with your doctor. Partnership with your own body. Blood pressure care works best when decisions are informed, questions are welcomed, and treatment is adjusted as life evolves. Changes in medication or strategy do not mean failure. They reflect thoughtful care.

It is also worth remembering why blood pressure control matters. The goal is not simply to improve numbers on a chart. The goal is to protect the heart from strain, the brain from stroke, the kidneys from silent damage, and the blood vessels from long-term injury. In doing so, blood pressure control protects independence, energy, and quality of life.

If there is one idea to hold onto, let it be this. High blood pressure does not need to dominate your thoughts or limit your life. When

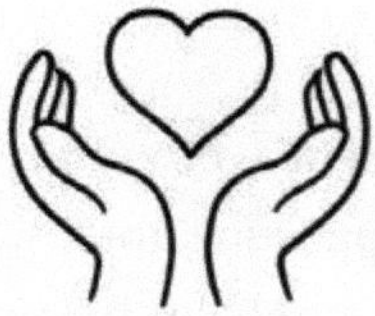

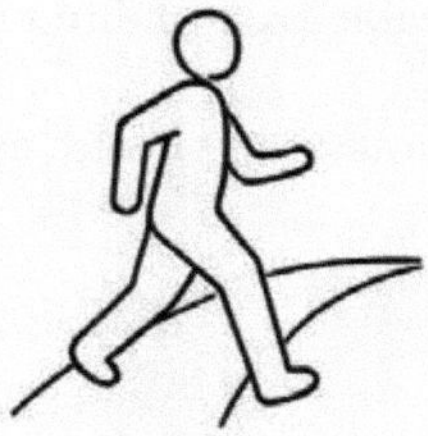

Tips for Living Well
with *High Blood Pressure*

understood and managed steadily, it becomes a background condition, monitored and controlled, rather than a constant source of worry.

As you close this book, take a moment to reflect on what you have learned and what feels most relevant to you. Choose one or two changes you can commit to comfortably. Build from there. Good health is not achieved in a single decision, but in the quiet accumulation of sensible choices over time.

With understanding, consistency, and patience, blood pressure can remain in a safe range for years to come, supporting not just longevity, but a fuller and more confident life. If this book has helped you feel more informed, more reassured, or more in control, then it has served its purpose. Carry that understanding forward, one day at a time. With patience and consistency, blood pressure can remain a manageable part of life rather than a source of worry.

I wish you steady health and quiet confidence in the journey ahead.

Thank You and Please Review the Book

Thank you for taking the time to read this book. I sincerely hope it has helped you understand your health a little more clearly and has given you practical, everyday steps you can follow with confidence.

If you found this book helpful, I would truly appreciate it if you could leave a brief and honest review. Even a few lines sharing your experience can make a meaningful difference. Your feedback helps other readers find reliable, trustworthy health information and supports them in making better decisions for themselves and their families.

Warm regards,

Dr Prabhat Das

Continue your Healthcare Journey

Good health is a journey, not a single step. It is not achieved in one day or with one book. That is why I created the "**Better Health with Dr Das** "series, with each book addressing a different common condition. If you would like easy, practical guidance on other everyday health concerns, you may wish to explore the rest of books in this series.

Books in this series:

- **A Doctor's Easy Guide to Understanding & Managing OBESITY.**
- **A Doctor's Easy Guide to Understanding & Managing HIGH BLOOD PRESSURE.**
- **Doctor, What DIET Is Best for Me? (Fad Diets, Myths, and What Really Works).**
  (being published)
- **The Truth About GLP-1 Medicines: A Doctor's Guide to Ozempic, Wegovy, Zepbound or Similar Medicines.**
  (being published)

Printed by Libri Plureos GmbH in Hamburg, Germany

9 781971 672366